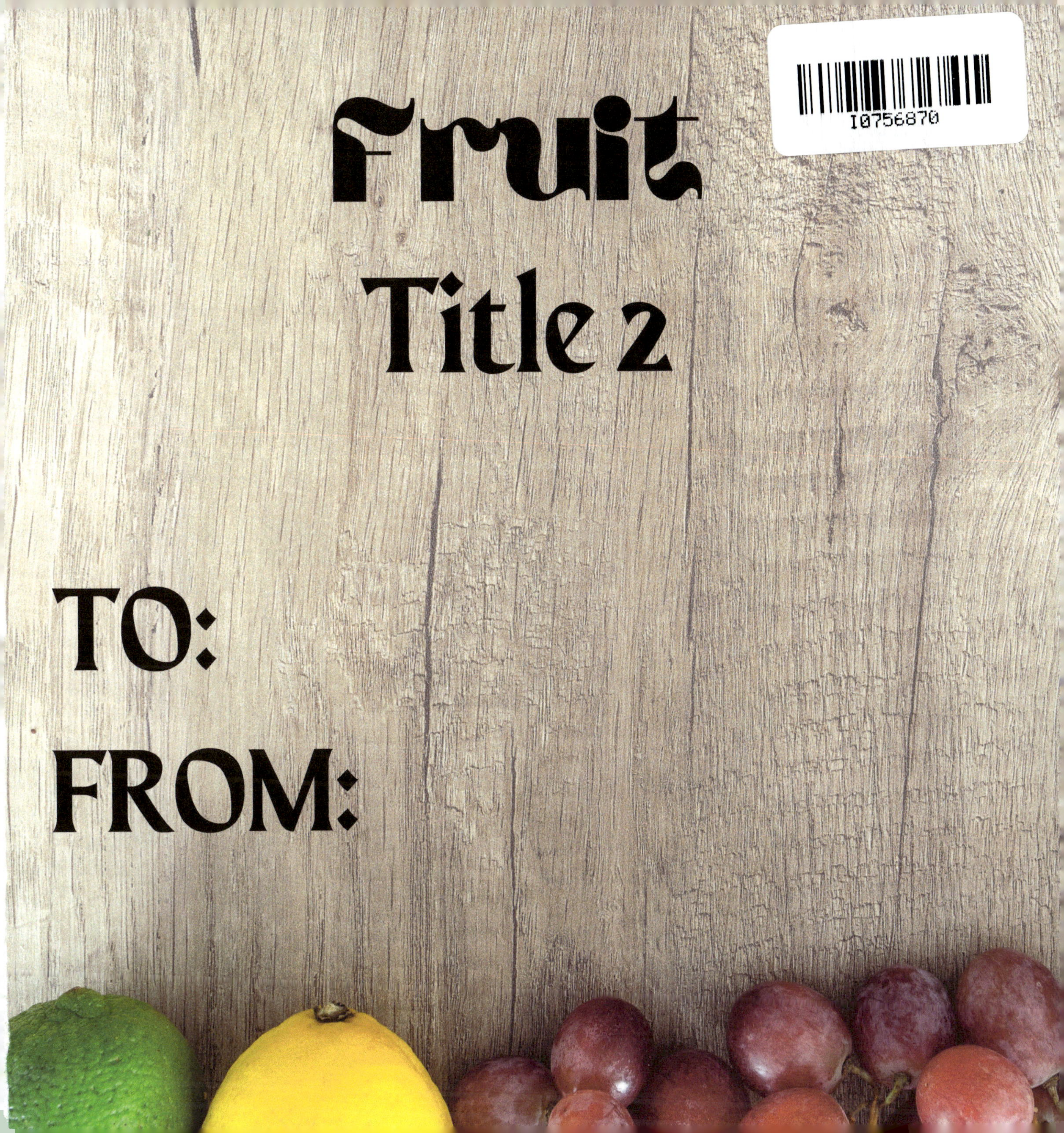

Fruit
Title 2
TO:
FROM:
I0756870

Cats are simply the most marvelous creatures. And if you're a dog owner, the world forgives you! :-)

I mean, cats have this indescribable way to fascinate everyone, even dogs. If you're lucky to have a cat in your world then you're truly blessed.

~ Joy Visante

NO ONE CAN REAP THE FRUIT BEFORE PLANTING THE TREES

LUIZ INACIO LULA DA SILVA

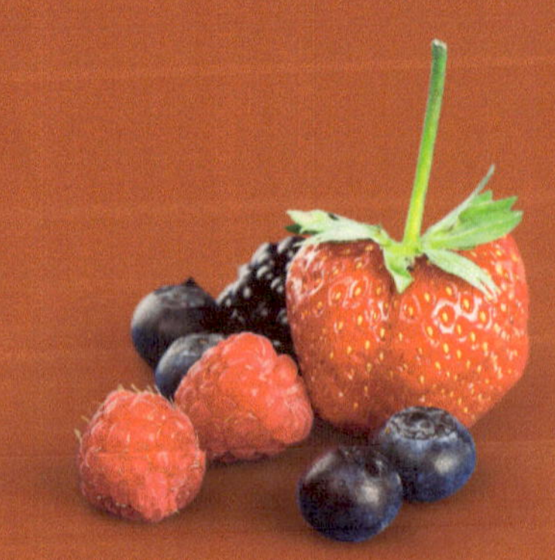

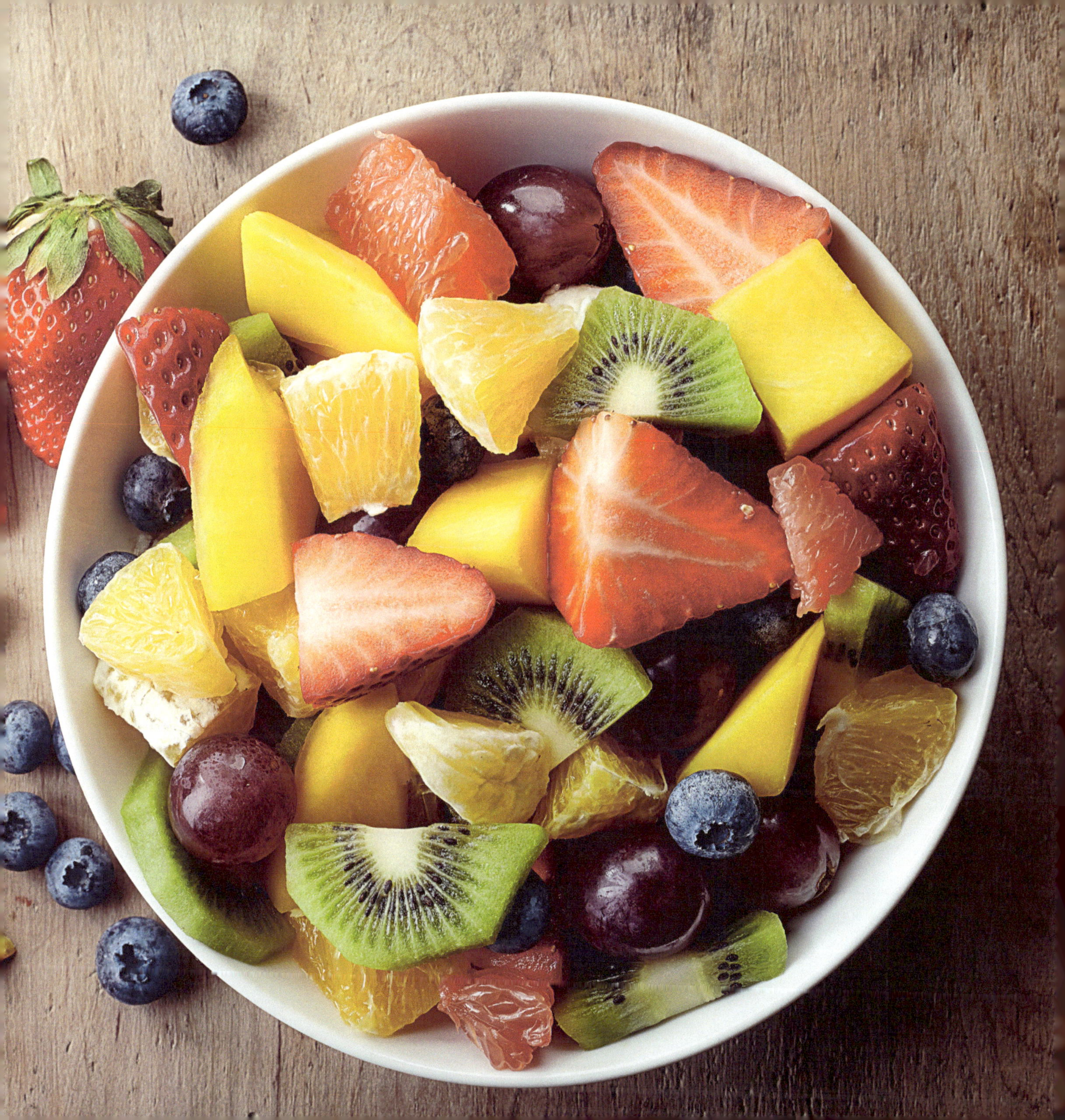

"WHEN LIFE GIVES YOU LEMONS, YOU SHOULD MAKE LEMONADE AND THEN TRY TO FIND SOMEONE WHOSE LIFE HAS GIVEN THEM VODKA, AND HAVE A PARTY."

RON WHITE

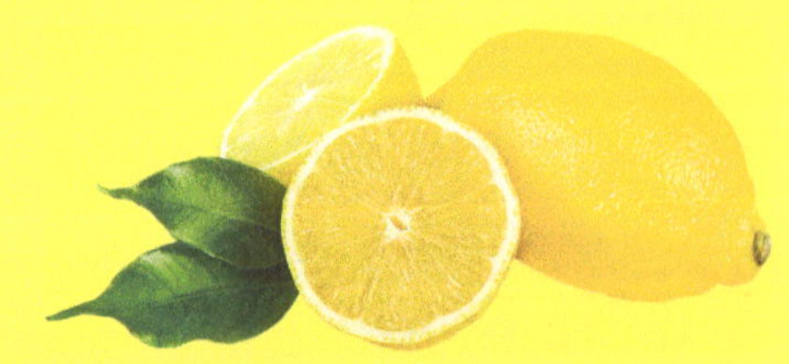

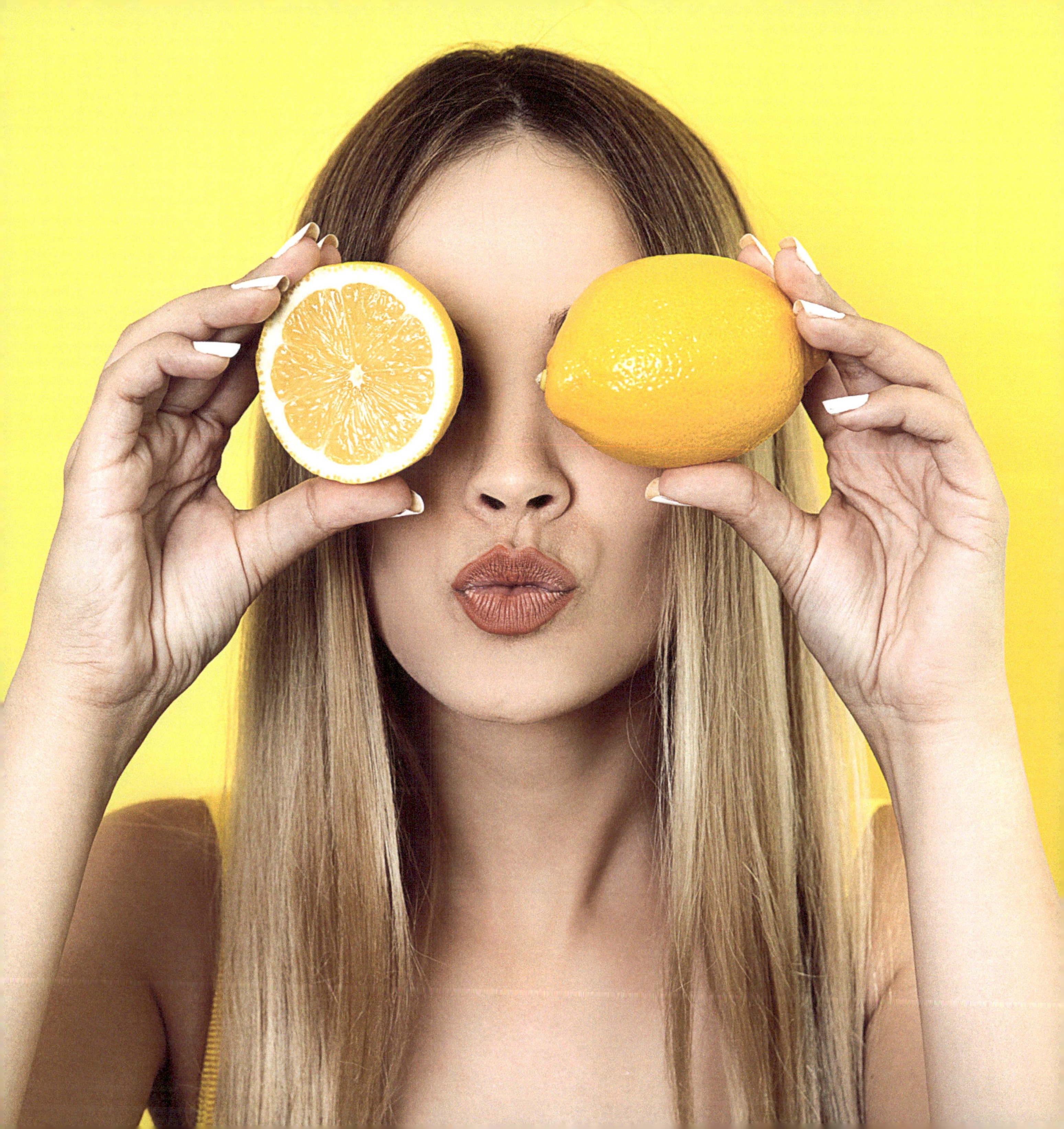

LIFE IS FULL OF BANANA SKINS. YOU SLIP, YOU CARRY ON

DAPHNE GUINNESS

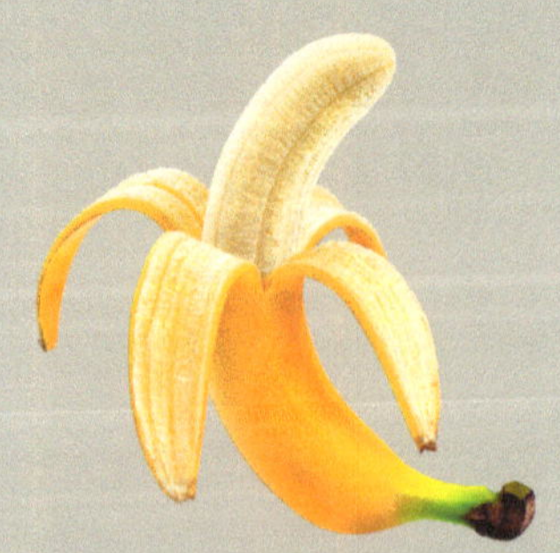

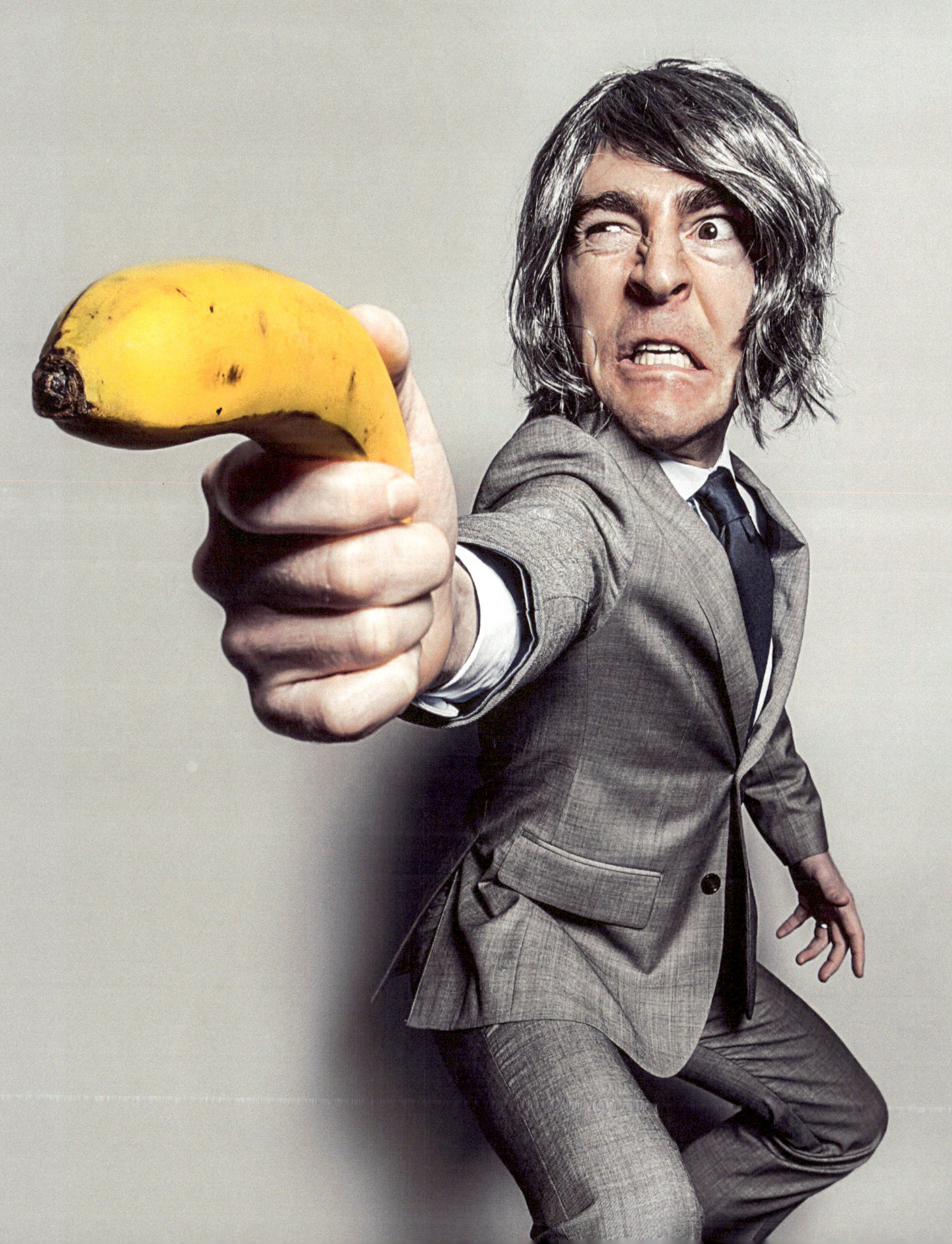

ANYONE CAN COUNT THE
NUMBER OF SEEDS IN AN
APPLE, BUT ONLY GOD
CAN COUNT THE NUMBER
OF APPLES IN A SEED

ROBERT H. SCHULLER

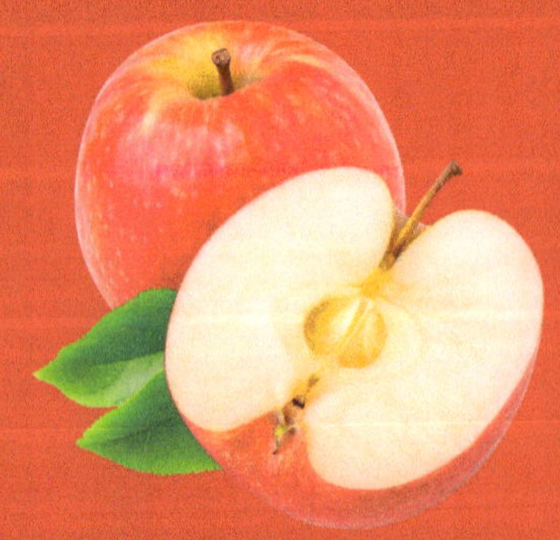

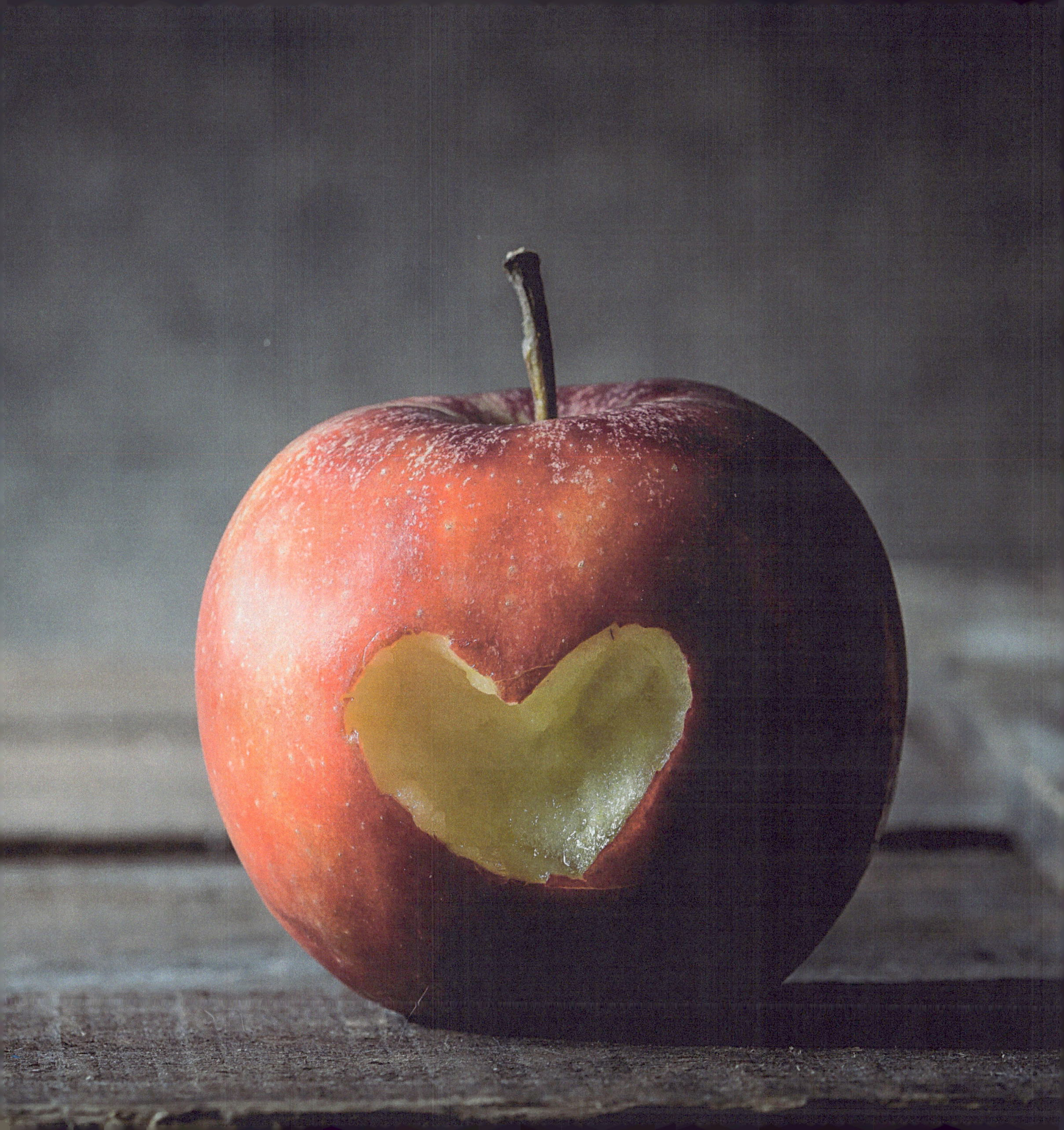

BE LIKE A PINEAPPLE. STAND TALL, WEAR A CROWN, AND BE SWEET ON THE INSIDE

KATHERINE GASKIN

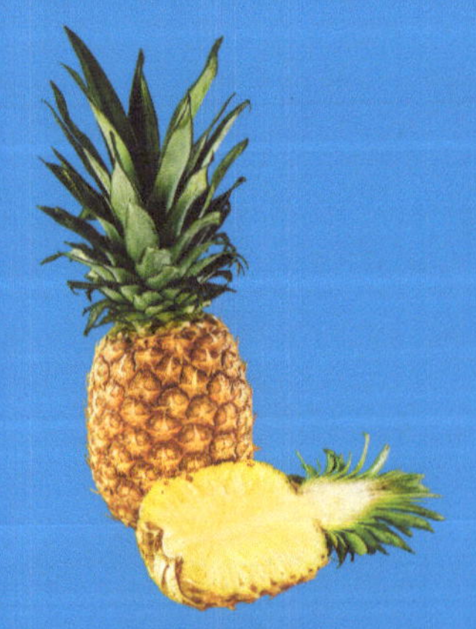

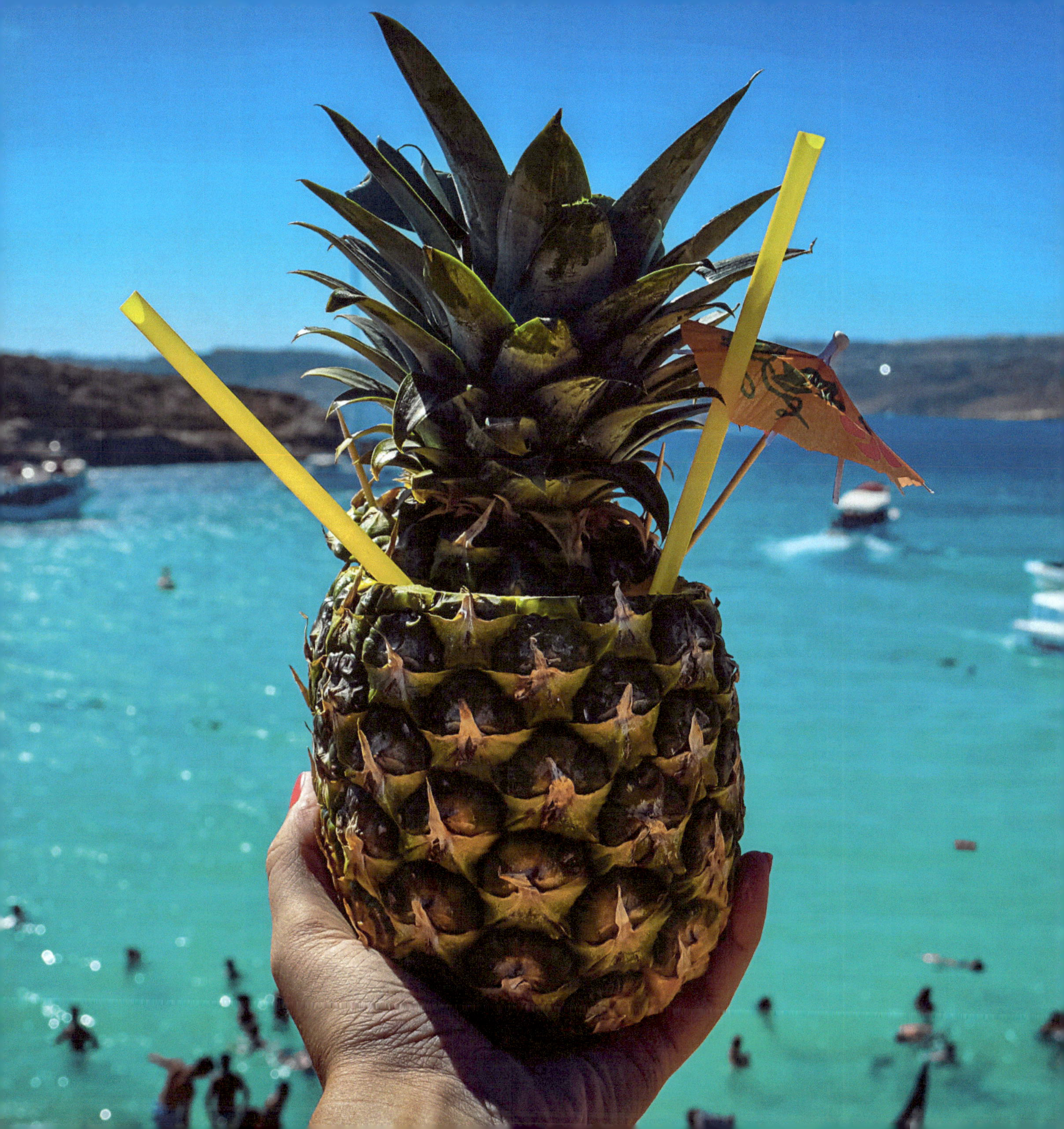

IN THE CHERRY BLOSSOM'S SHADE THERE'S NO SUCH THING AS A STRANGER.

KOBAYASHI ISSA

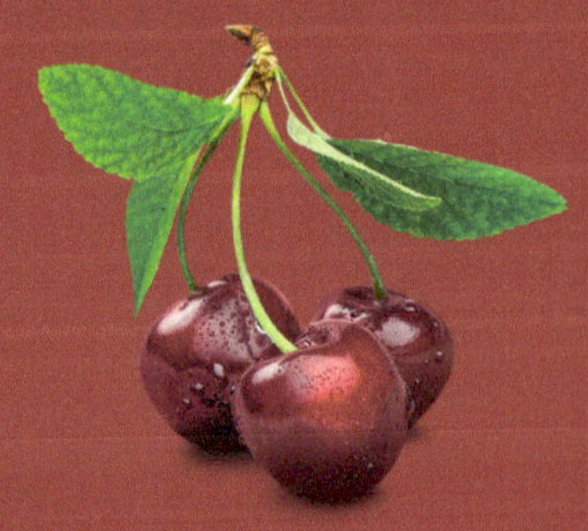

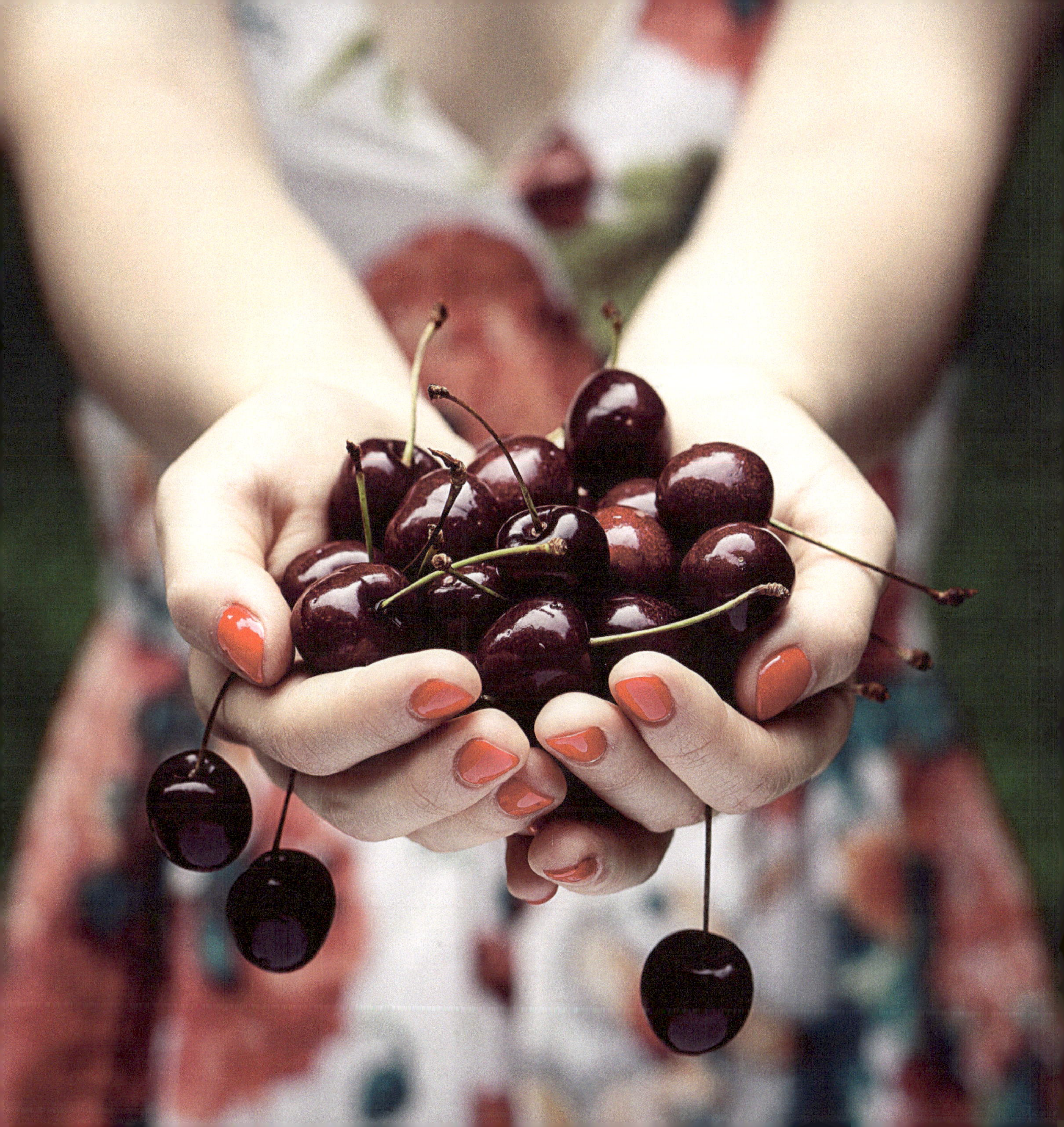

AND THE FRUITS WILL OUTDO WHAT THE FLOWERS HAVE PROMISED.

FRANÇOIS DE MALHERBE

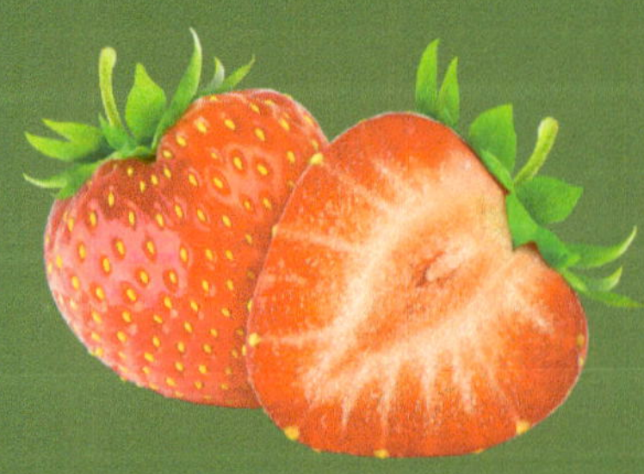

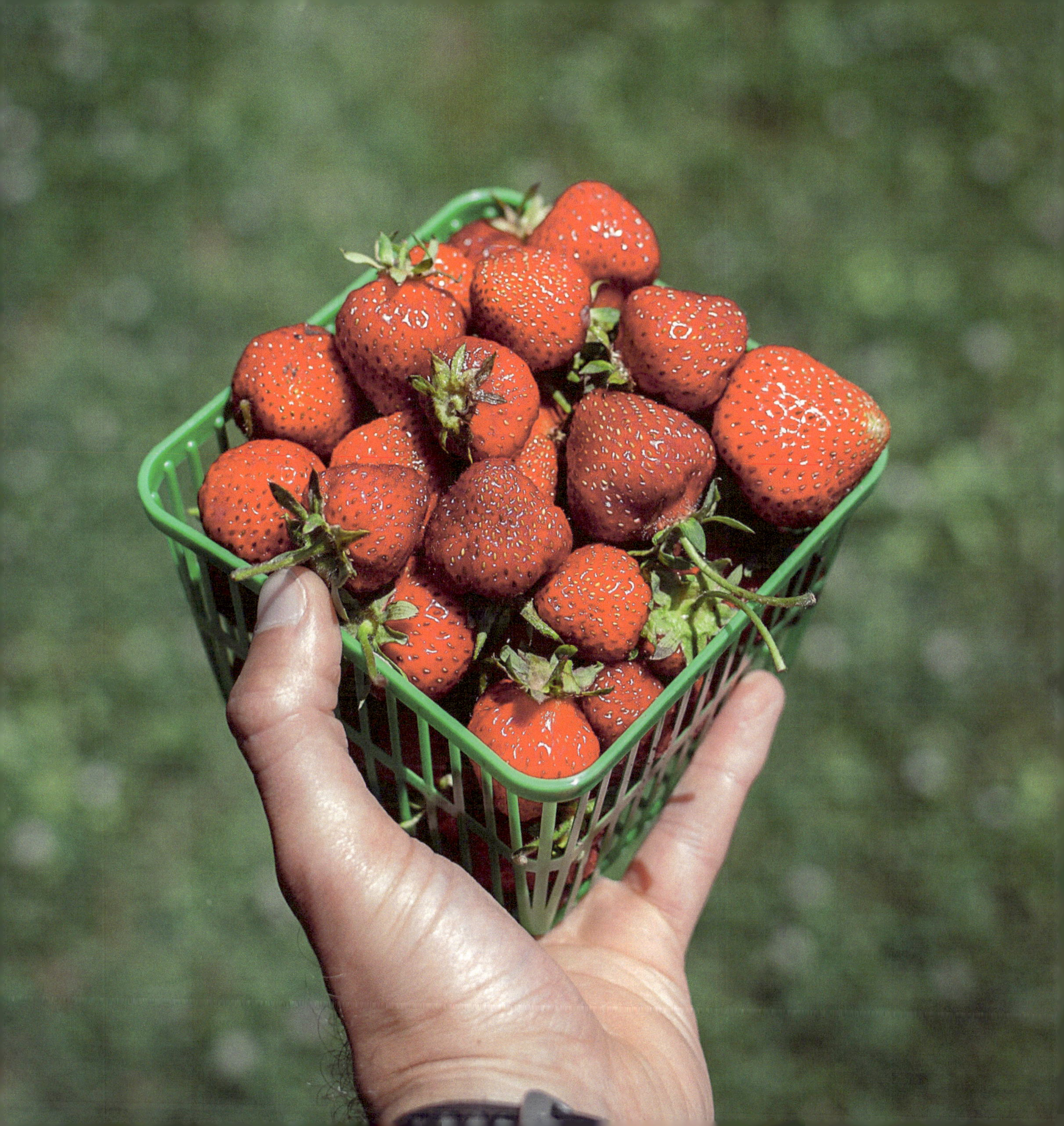

WHILE FORBIDDEN FRUIT IS SAID TO TASTE SWEETER, IT USUALLY SPOILS FASTER.

ABIGAIL VAN BUREN

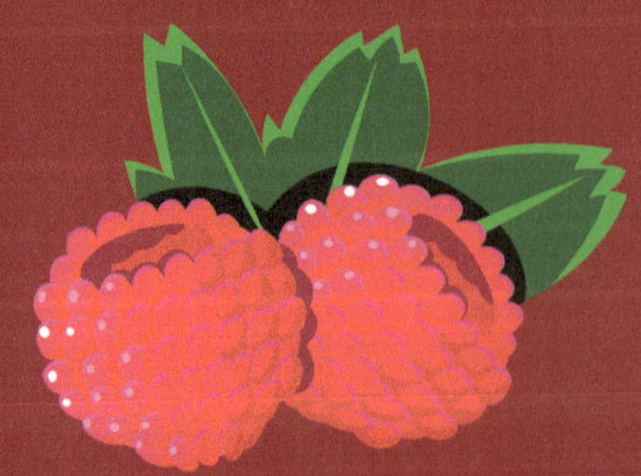

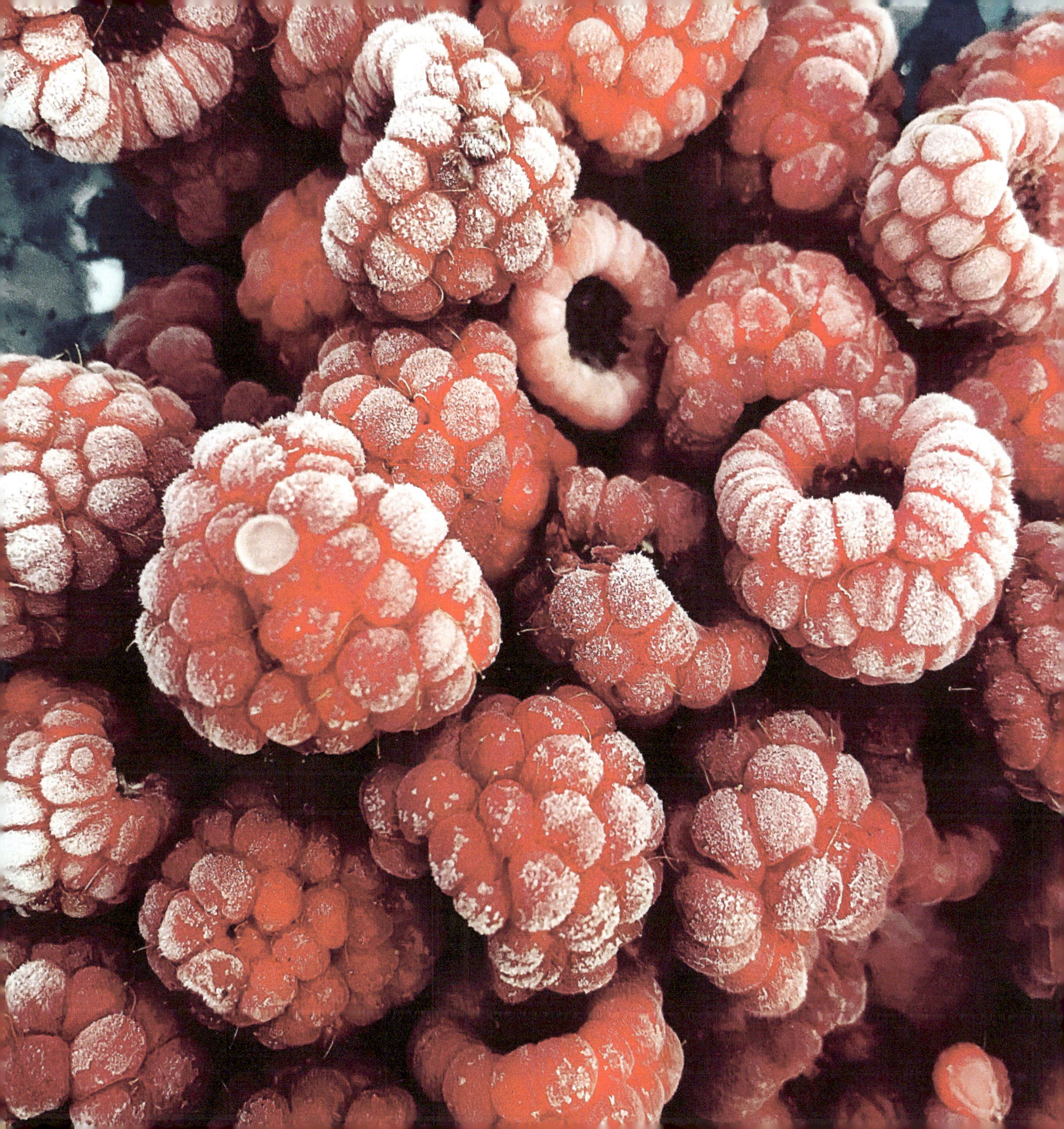

TASTE EVERY FRUIT OF EVERY TREE IN THE GARDEN AT LEAST ONCE. IT IS AN INSULT TO CREATION NOT TO EXPERIENCE IT FULLY. TEMPERANCE IS WICKEDNESS.

STEPHEN FRY

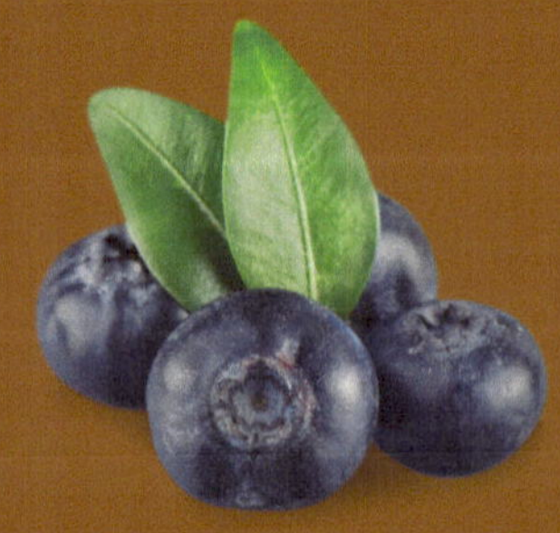

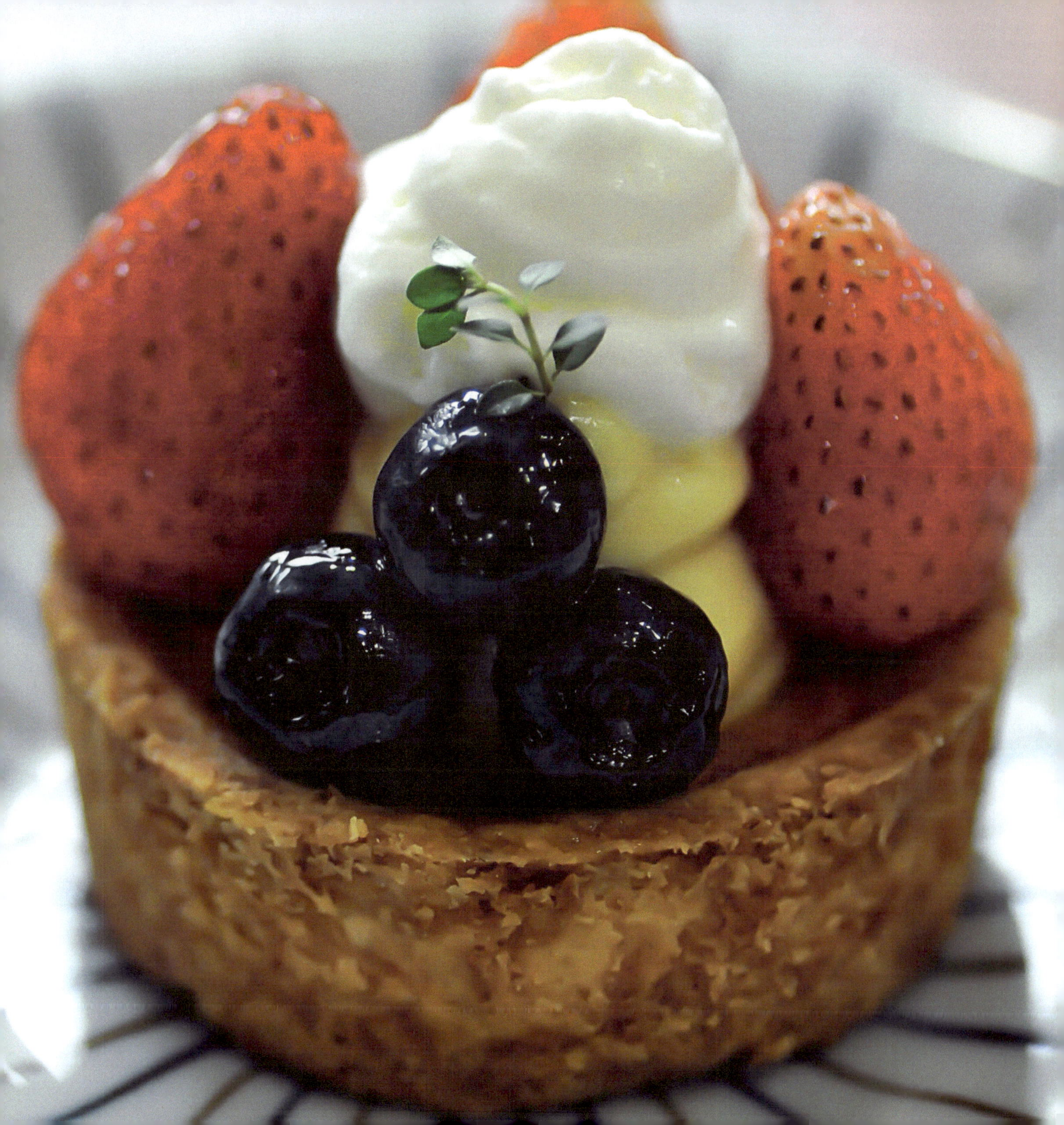

FORBIDDEN FRUIT TASTES SWEET, BUT ITS AFTERTASTE IS BITTER.

JOHN F. KENNEDY

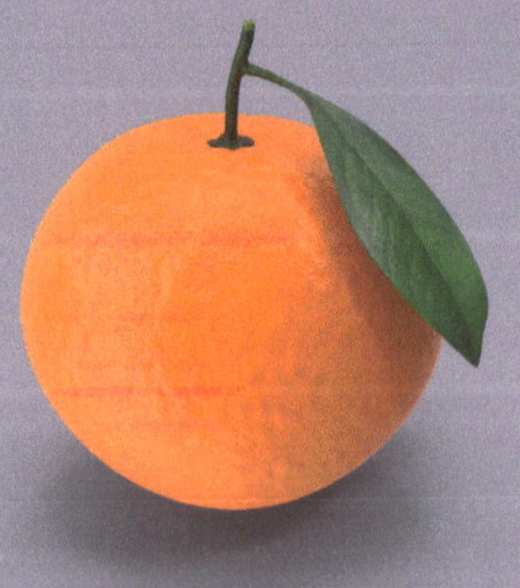

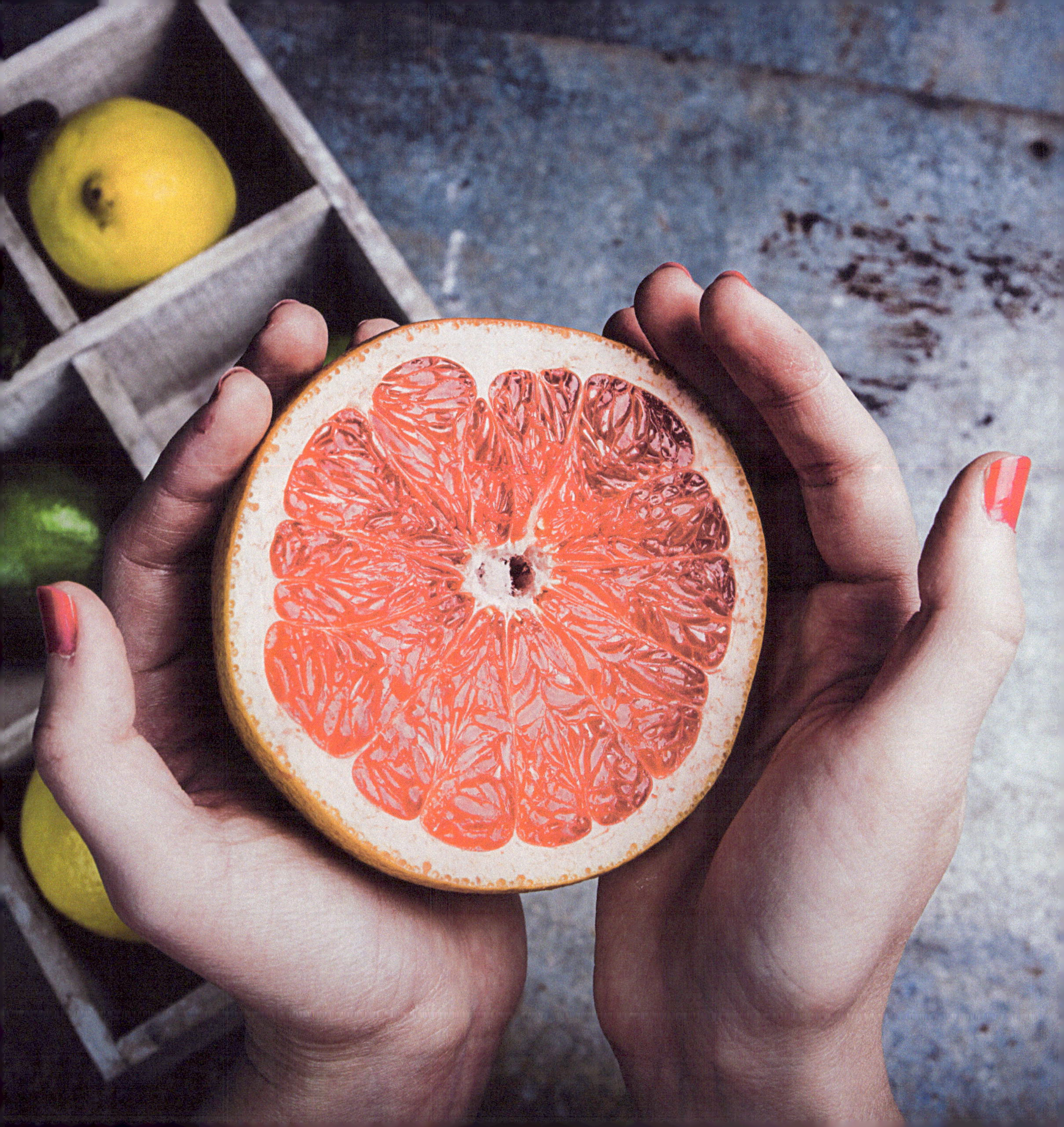

FRUITS THAT BLOSSOM FIRST WILL FIRST BE RIPE.

WILLIAM SHAKESPEARE

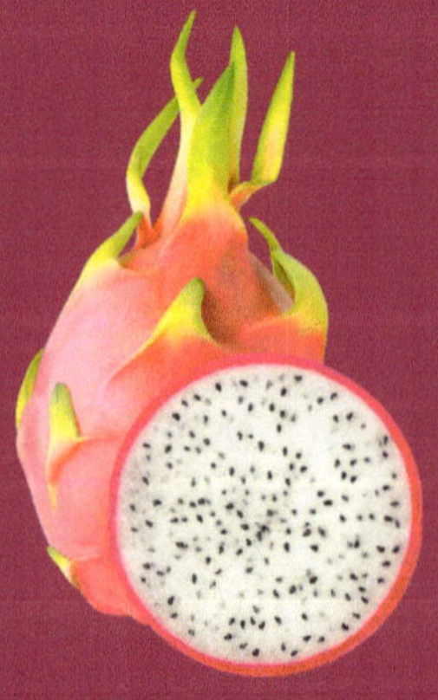

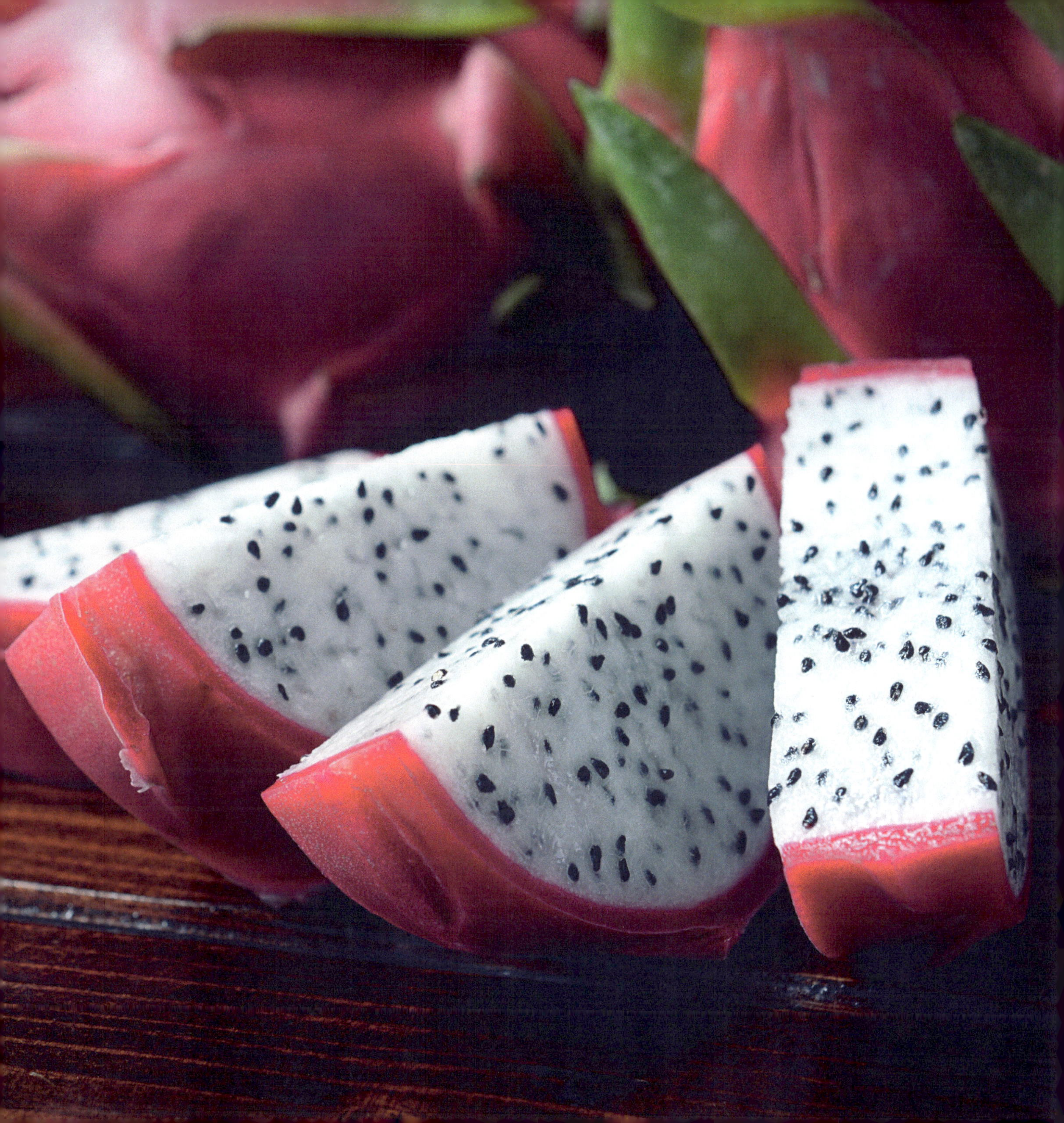

THE WEAKEST KIND OF FRUIT DROPS EARLIEST TO THE GROUND.

WILLIAM SHAKESPEARE

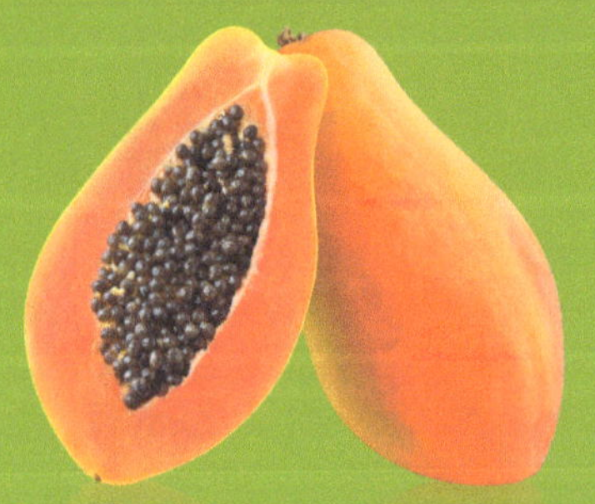

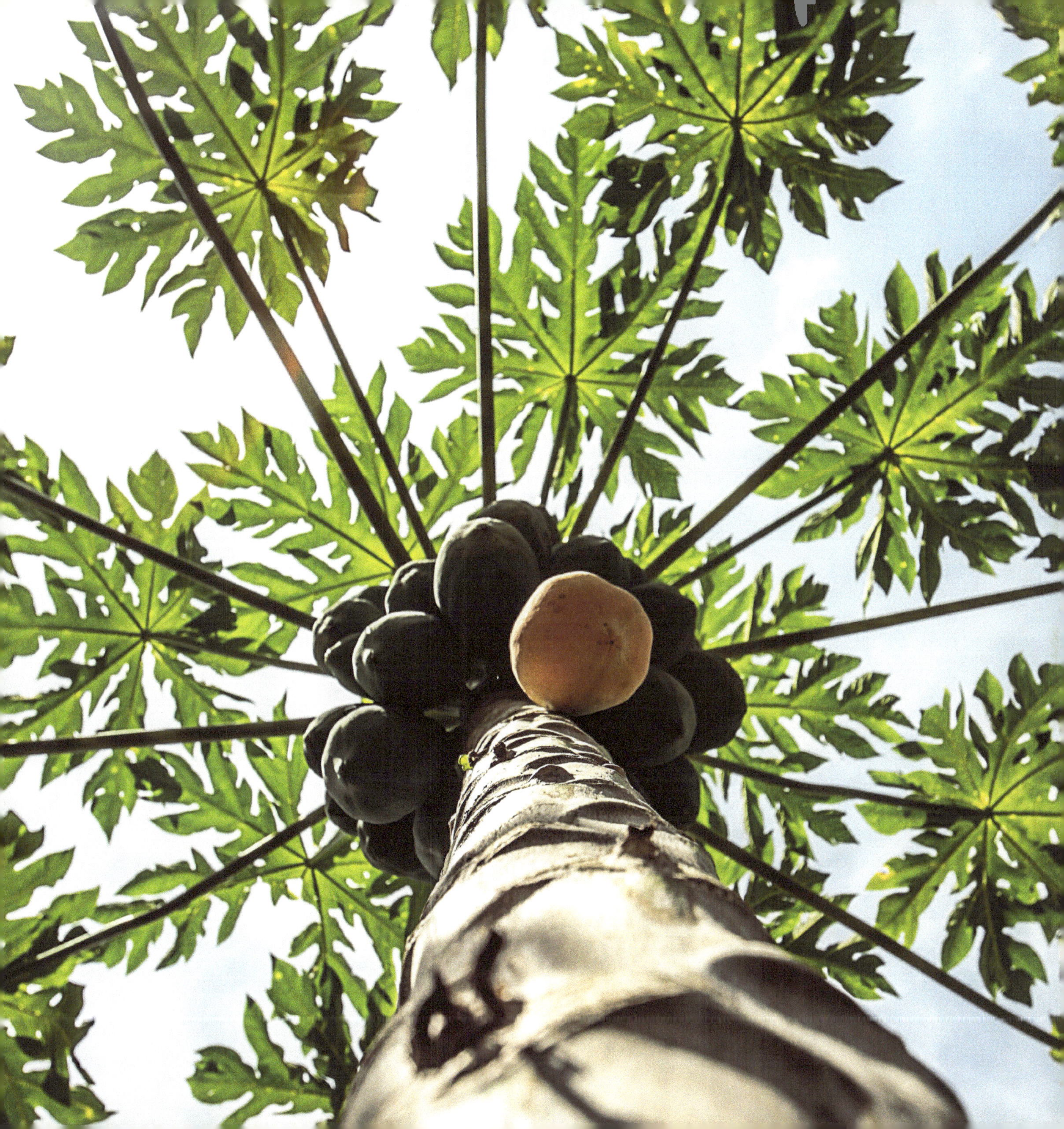

ALL FRUIT GROWS THROUGH ABIDING, NOT STRIVING.

BILL JOHNSON

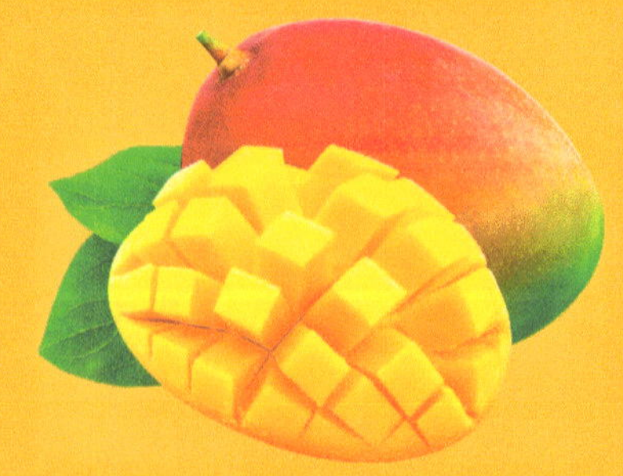

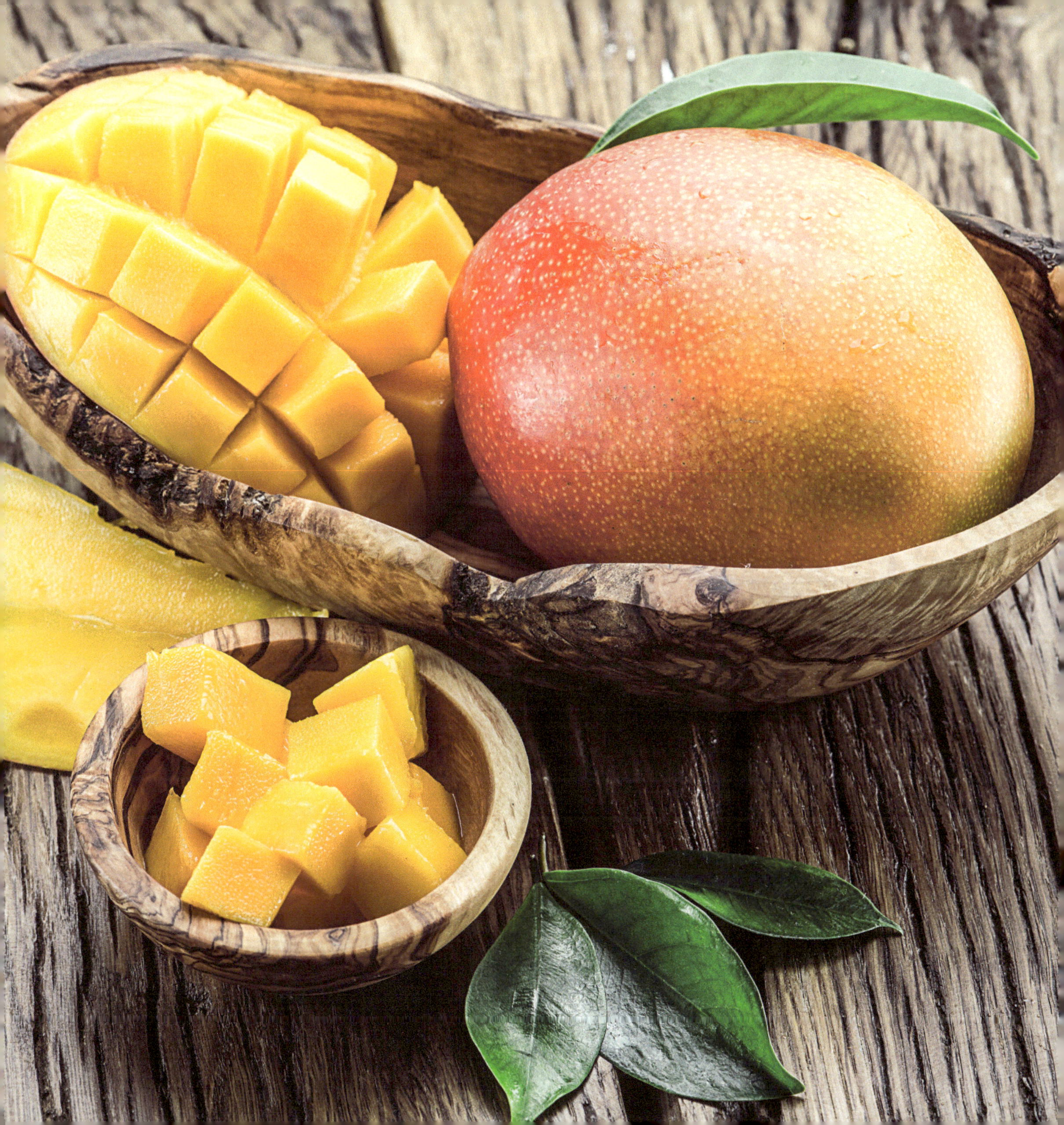

IF THERE IS A FRUIT THAT CAN BE EATEN RAW, IT IS BEAUTY

ALPHONSE KARR

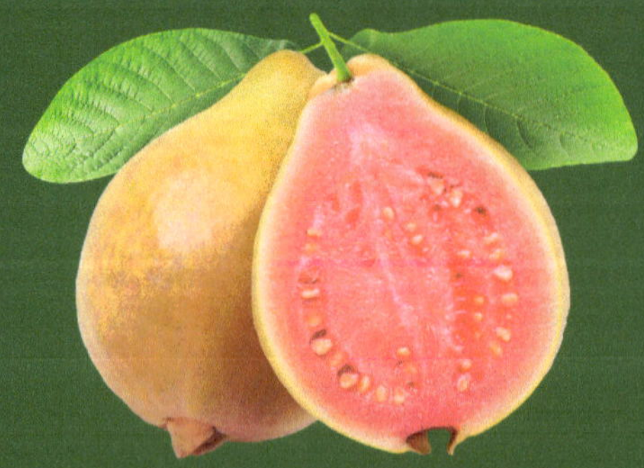

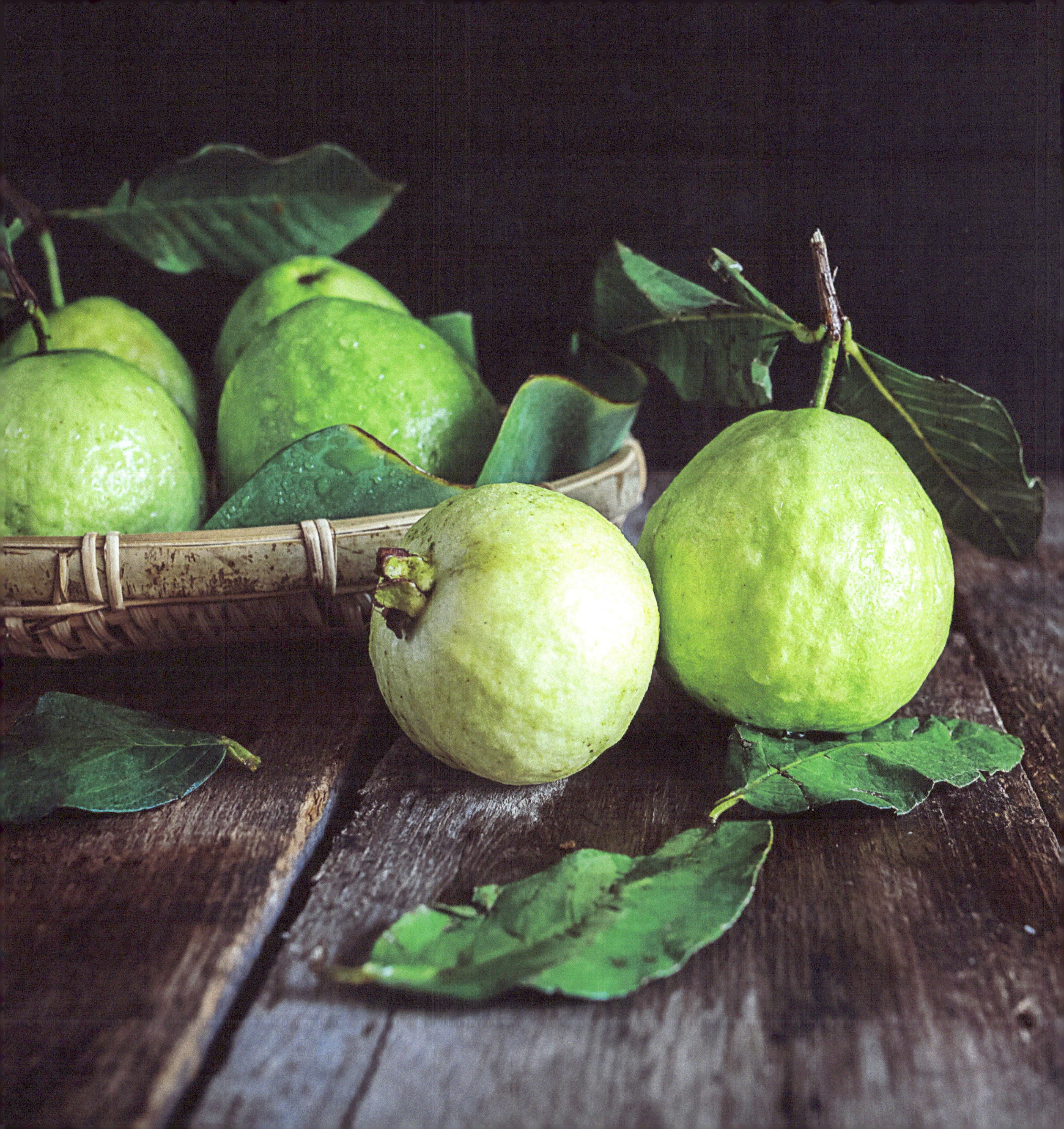

THERE IS NO FRUIT WHICH IS NOT BITTER BEFORE IT IS RIPE

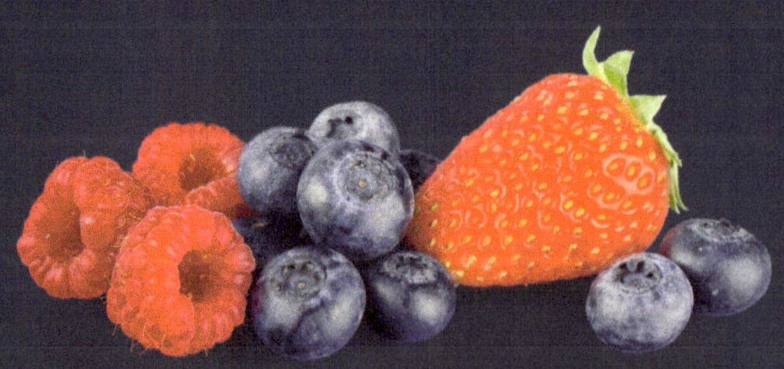

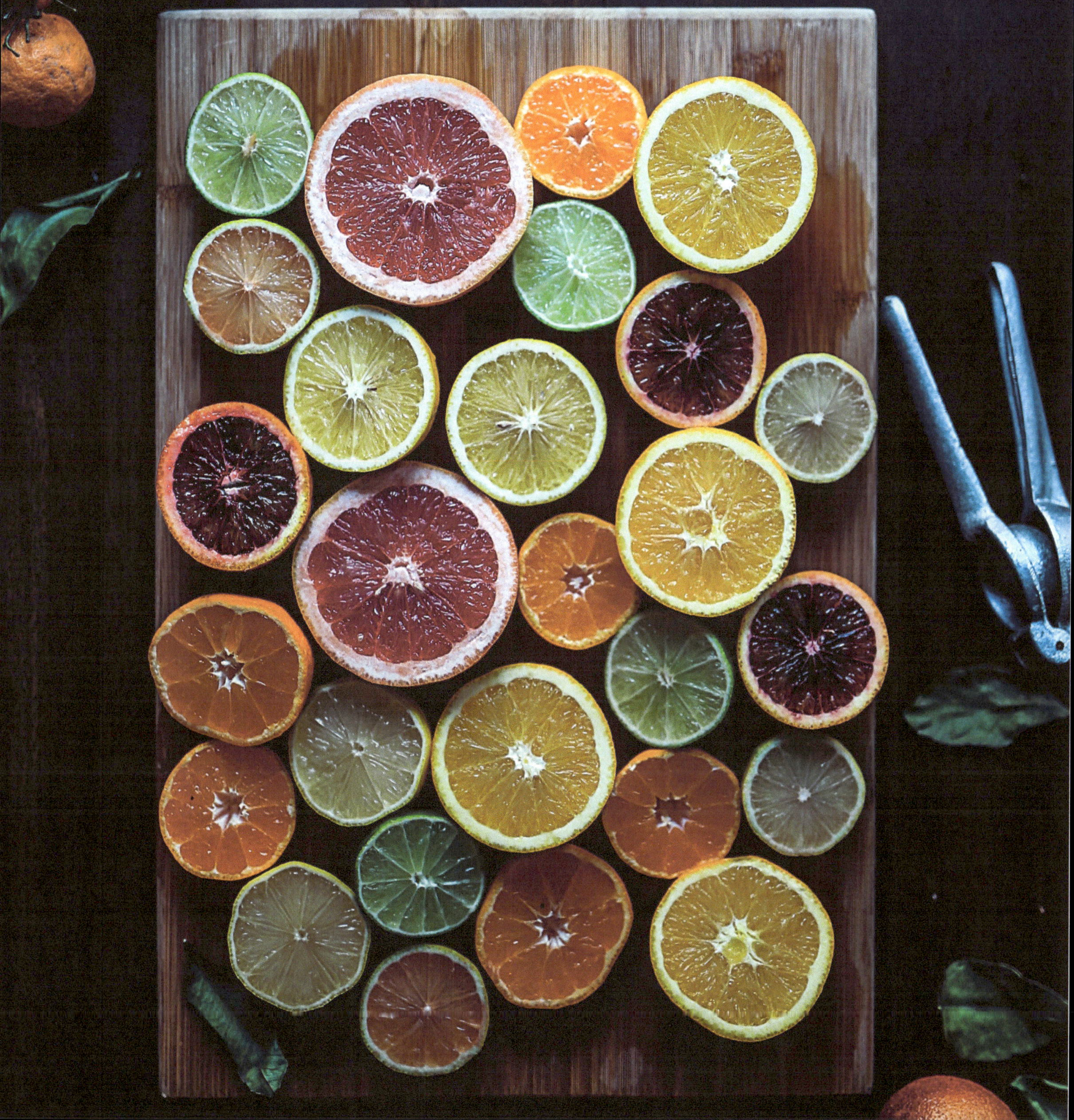

FRUIT FORCED IS NEVER HALF SO SWEET / AS THAT COMES QUITE IN SEASON.

CAROLINE ANNE SOUTHEY

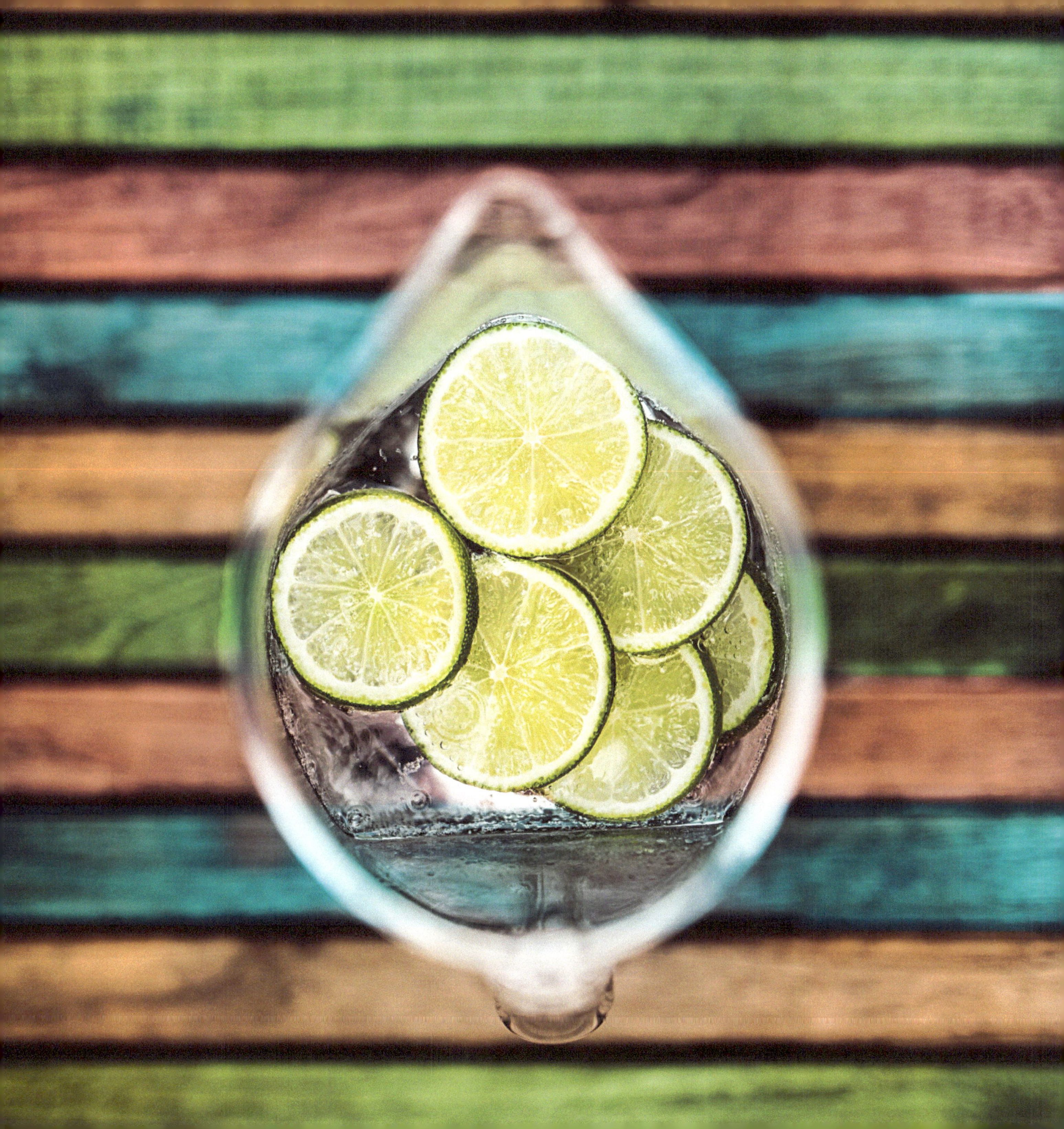

THE FRUIT DERIVED FROM LABOR IS THE SWEETEST OF PLEASURES

LUC DE CLAPIERS

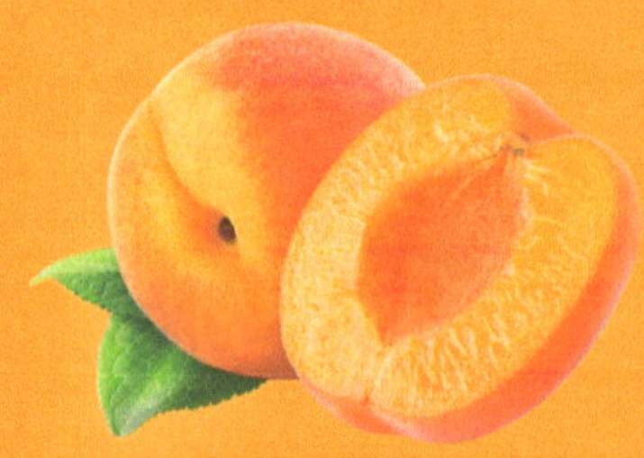

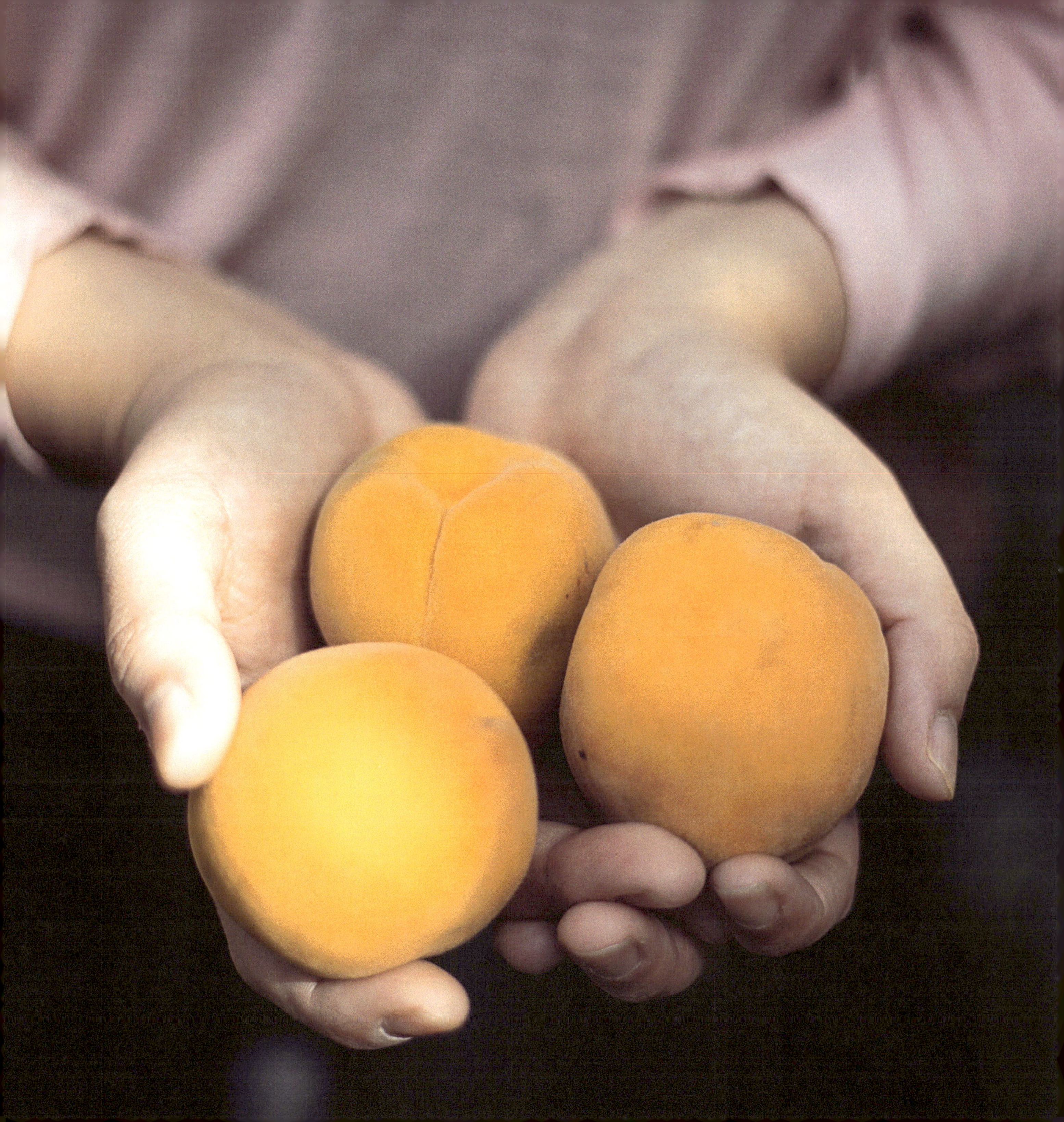

THE FRUIT OF YOUR OWN HARD WORK IS THE SWEETEST.

DEEPIKA PADUKONE

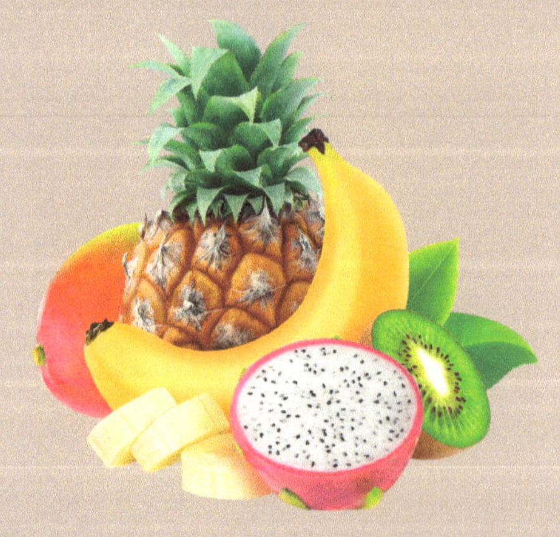